Really Healthy

Gluten Free Living

How to heal your gut
with a healthy gluten free diet

Includes 32 healthy gluten free recipes

Janet Matthews Dip ION

CONTENTS

ᘏᘉᘄ

PREFACE

☙❧

Celiac Disease is a debilitating disease that can cause significant damage to the gut if it is not diagnosed and addressed. Other health conditions such as Gluten Intolerance, a milder condition than celiac disease, can also cause damage to the gut and result in chronic illness.

People who have been diagnosed with Celiac Disease and those with Gluten Intolerance need to be on a gluten free diet, but what seems to becoming more evident is that although a gluten free diet prevents further damage from occurring, it may not be enough to heal the damage already done to the gut.

Gluten is known to damage the lining of the gut causing allergies and digestive problems. It also adversely affects the efficacy of the immune system.

Research from the University of Chicago found that the small intestines of up to 60% of adults with Celiac Disease will never completely heal if the adherence to the diet is less than optimal.

In 2009 a study in the Journal of Alimentary Pharmacology and Therapeutics found that out of 465 celiac patients who had been on a gluten free diet for 16 months, the gut tissue had only normalized in 8% of the patients. In addition 65% of the patients were still suffering from inflammation in the gut.

In 2002 another study (in the same journal) of 30 adults who had Celiac Disease confirmed that after 10 years on a gluten free diet, 56% had a poor vitamin status. This would seem to imply that their digestive systems were not absorbing the nutrients they were consuming.

According to a study involving 188 people on gluten free diets, the University of Chicago Celiac Disease Centre reported that after 2 years on a gluten free diet 81% had gained weight.

These results would certainly beg the question as to whether a gluten free diet is as healthy as we are led to believe or is there something intrinsically wrong with the way people are interpreting this diet.

The recent increase in the diagnosis of Celiac Disease and Gluten Intolerance has resulted in a huge increase in gluten free products appearing in our health food stores and supermarkets. In many ways these gluten free products are lulling us into a false sense of security. A large number of these products have lost sight of the meaning of what constitutes a healthy diet and have failed to take into account the requirements of the sufferers who need to heal the damage done by the gluten. The research results have indicated that a gluten free diet isn't enough and isn't producing the healing results that we are looking for. It is also my opinion that the gluten free product industry isn't helping their cause.

Unfortunately the majority of us want to find the easiest option to solve our problems, the one that challenges us the least. Of course it is possible to do that and you may well get a quick fix, but if you want real lasting results you may need to open yourself up to a bigger challenge and experience for yourself whether you think it was worth it.

WHY I HAVE WRITTEN THIS BOOK?

∝≫

My interest in the affects of gluten on our health came about because of my own health story. For many years I have suffered from intestinal bloating, headaches, occasional feelings of an inflamed gut and occasional bouts of irritable bowel syndrome. I had never really been able to get to the bottom of it. Due to the fact that I suffered from some fungal type infections, I had thought initially that I might have had Candida Albicans, a parasitic fungal overgrowth that resides in the intestine and which can become systemic (affects other systems of the body). Although I had some relief from following an anti candida regime it didn't solve the problem completely and I was still left with many unanswered questions

In 2009 after several years of trying to find the cause of my condition, I consulted a clinical nutritionist who advised me to invest in a variety of tests to see if we could ascertain why I was suffering from these seemingly unexplained health issues.

The diagnosis came back that I was gluten intolerant. I had several foods I was mildly and moderately intolerant to, there was evidence of yeast in my gut and I had 3 parasites. I did not in fact have Candida Albicans as I had suspected but the parasites and the yeast went a long way to explain why I had been suffering from these symptoms and had been unable to eradicate them. In addition to this I had a leaky gut (holes in the lining of the gut wall) and low levels of good bacteria in my gut. As we shall see when I discuss this later in the book all of these conditions are closely linked and can be brought together to complete the symptom picture

Being diagnosed with Celiac Disease or Gluten Intolerance puts many people into a state of panic as they envisage many of their favorite foods disappearing over the horizon. Bread, pasta, cakes and biscuits are the main stay of many people's diet and the first thing a newly diagnosed sufferer looks for is the gluten free alternatives. But there is more to recovering from Celiac Disease or Gluten Intolerance than simply finding gluten free alternatives.

I am about to explore what constitutes a **Really Healthy Gluten Free Diet**, look at ways you can start to heal your gut to work towards a full recovery, and in doing so clear up the many misconceptions surrounding these conditions. You may even find that other niggling health conditions clear up as well as a result of the changes you make to your diet.

CHAPTER 1
WHAT IS GLUTEN

☙

Gluten is a protein made up of two peptides - gliadin and glutenin. It is what causes dough to have its elastic properties and gives the finished bread product its structure and shape. Very strong wheat bread flours have a high gluten content as giving the bread a strong structure is an important component of successful bread making. However cake flour is generally a weaker gluten flour as we want our cakes to be light and spongy and a strong structure isn't what we are after.

Gliadin is a prolamine, a toxic protein that is incredibly difficult for humans to digest. The human gut is not able to break them down into small enough particles for absorption. As a result they can cause severe damage to the lining of the gut wall and subsequent gut inflammation.

Glutenin is responsible for keeping bread raised and light in texture. However it is also responsible for the addictive quality of the food, and can result in cravings and addictive behavior.

WHAT IS CELIAC DISEASE?

It is not so long ago that it was believed that a gluten free diet applied only to those diagnosed with celiac disease, a chronic condition classified as an auto immune disease. The body's immune system begins to attack itself when the sufferer eats any food containing gluten. Even the smallest quantities of gluten can affect the celiac causing damage and inflammation to the lining of the gut wall. Cilia that line the gut stand upright and aid the absorption of food, in a celiac the cilia have been flattened, which consequently affects the absorption of food. If viewed long term we can see that poor absorption of food is going to affect the overall health of the person with celiac disease, and so prompt action is required as soon as a diagnosis has been received. The only way to effectively treat this disease is to eliminate gluten completely from the diet and to work towards restoring the integrity of the gut wall.

It is also important for the celiac to ensure that there is no cross contamination of gluten in their kitchen which involves rigorous care and attention, especially when sharing the kitchen with a non celiac.

Symptoms of Celiac Disease are many and varied. They include:

- Diarrhea and/or constipation, which is often accompanied by excessive wind.
- Gastrointestinal symptoms including: nausea, vomiting, bloating, cramping and other stomach pain.
- Ulcers in the mouth.
- Alopecia (hair loss).
- Depression.
- Possible weight loss.
- Poor bone density due poor absorption of calcium.
- Unexplained chronic tiredness .
- Type 1 diabetes is particularly prevalent amongst celiac.
- Problems with fertility and an increased possibility of miscarriage.

Although the list of symptoms may appear to be quite depressing to a newly diagnosed celiac, the good news is it can be treated, and the first line of defense is to embark on a healthy gluten free diet. As soon as gluten is eliminated the gut wall has the chance to start to recover and repair itself. However full healing may not be as simple as eliminating gluten, especially if you have been suffering for some time, as there are also other things that need to be done in order to heal the gut wall as we shall discover.

If you suspect that you may have celiac disease then your doctor can do a test. If the test comes back positive then apart from finding out as much as you can about healing your gut and healthy gluten free diets, no more tests should be necessary. However if the test comes back negative you may wish to have a test done privately, as I did, to ascertain if you have a gluten intolerance.

WHAT IS GLUTEN INTOLERANCE?

Gluten Intolerance has similar, though often less severe, symptoms than Celiac Disease. Despite the fact that it is not thought to involve the immune system in the same way as Celiac Disease, it can cause quite serious damage to the lining of the gut wall. This can cause leaky gut syndrome, (discussed in detail in chapter 4) which in turn causes various allergies and intolerances to other foods. A person who is gluten sensitive is less likely to have an immediate symptom as a result of eating gluten, although this is not always the case, as it depends on the severity of the intolerance. The results, however, are just as damaging to the gut over time and many of the symptoms listed above for the celiac apply to those who are gluten sensitive as well.

It is thought that far more people than those diagnosed are actually sensitive to gluten and are damaging the delicate lining of the gut without realizing it. But as I mentioned earlier the only way to get a diagnosis of gluten sensitivity is to pay for a test to be done privately under the guidance of a qualified clinical nutritionist who can help you to understand the results and offer you support.

If, as has been suggested, approximately 1% of the population have been diagnosed with celiac disease then it is fair to presume that the true figure may be in excess of that as it is likely that there are many people who are still undiagnosed. If we add to that the number of people who have a gluten intolerance or who are unable to tolerate wheat, then the percentage starts to rise even more. With that in mind it is important for all of us to educate ourselves regarding gluten free diets and to become more aware of the foods that we buy on a regular basis that contain gluten, especially those that have hidden gluten that we have previously been unaware of.

Chapter 2
What To Do When You Have Been Diagnosed With Celiac Disease Or Gluten Intolerance

❀

It would seem to me that there are 3 main issues here that need to be addressed to ensure that a full recovery is achieved:

1. Understand that after the initial diagnosis you need to eliminate gluten completely from your diet and acquire an understanding what constitutes a healthy gluten free diet

2. Be aware of the damage that gluten has done to your gut leading to leaky gut syndrome, understanding how this impacts on your health and knowing what you need to do to repair the holes in your gut to enable you to achieve a full recovery

3. To complete the process you need to re populate the gut with good bacteria and subsequently improve digestion and absorption and to ultimately restore your immune system to full strength

In most instances the person diagnosed will simply eliminate the gluten without giving any thought to repairing the damaged gut, mainly because they are not aware that this is a necessary part of the healing and also because they don't know how to go about it.

A full recovery will occur much sooner if all of these issues are dealt with. If the gut wall is damaged, the good bacteria will have nothing to hold on to so it is important to attend to all of these issues from the onset.

Now we will take a more detailed look at how to go about this.

CHAPTER 3
ELIMINATING GLUTEN FROM THE DIET

First of all you need to be aware of which foods contain gluten. Regarding foods that naturally contain gluten it is a matter of remembering what they are. It will help enormously if you remove any you may already have from your store cupboard. You may find this difficult to do initially but it will undoubtedly help you in the long run. It goes without saying that these foods should not appear on your future shopping lists!

FOODS THAT CONTAIN GLUTEN

Barley
Bulgur wheat
Breakfast cereals containing wheat and oats
Cereal based protein
Couscous
Durum wheat used in pasta
Kamut
Malt
Oats (rolled. Porridge, jumbo)
Oat bran } There is a divergence of opinion regarding oats.
Oatmeal } My advice is only to buy oats that state they are gluten free as they are often milled on the same site as wheat products
Pearl barley
Rye

Semolina
Spelt
Triticale (a mixture of wheat and rye)
Vegetable gum
Whole wheat
Wheat bran
Wheat germ

FOODS WITH HIDDEN GLUTEN

These foods may contain hidden gluten. Most of these products are available gluten free but you need to read the labels

Baking powder
Battered products and products covered in breadcrumbs
Beer and lager (made from grain)
Corn tortillas (most have wheat flour as well)
Gravy mixes and other seasoning mixes
Mustard powder
Processed meats such as sausages
Salad dressings and mayonnaise
Soups – may have flour to thicken or contain pearl barley
Soy sauce
Stock cubes and stock powder
Tablets that contain fillers
White pepper

These are just a few examples of foods you need to check. Most manufactured foods now say if they are gluten free. If it doesn't say gluten free then you need to check for yourself before purchasing.

GLUTEN FREE FOODS

There are plenty of healthy, natural foods for you to choose from that are gluten free including:

Meat
Fish
Eggs
Dairy products (milk, cheese, butter, cream, natural yoghurt, crème fraiche)
All fresh fruit and vegetables

Sprouted beans seeds, and lentils
Dried pulses (peas beans and lentils)
Nuts and seeds
Tamari (soy) sauce
Healthy oils such as extra virgin olive oil and coconut oil for cooking and sunflower for dressings
Vinegar and homemade salad dressings
Fresh herbs and spices

ALTERNATIVE GRAINS

As grains are the main area of difficulty for those who have to avoid gluten I will list the alternative grains that you can use that do not contain gluten and give you a brief description of their nutritional value. Most of them can be used as flour alternatives and are generally part of a flour blend, depending on whether they are for bread or other baking recipes

I would like to add here that for some people gluten free grains can also be problematic particularly in the early stages of the healing and it may be necessary initially to eliminate all grains for a short amount of time. This allows the gut to recover and start the healing process without being challenged by these grains. Undigested carbohydrates will only serve to exacerbate any inflammation in the gut and therefore will prevent any real healing from taking place.

However for those who may wish to use the alternative grains here is the list

Amaranth - This gluten free grain is an excellent source of protein, in particular the amino acid lysine, which is why amaranth is considered to be of a high "biological value". It also contains magnesium, calcium, iron and fiber. You can also pop amaranth like popcorn.

Brown Rice – Brown rice is a gluten free grain. It contains magnesium, B vitamins, iron and fiber. It is important to be aware that most of the nutritional value is removed when the rice is hulled and polished (when it becomes white rice) White rice is mainly pure carbohydrate – though some nutrients maybe added back in. Brown rice is by far the better option and can be bought as rice, flour, pasta and commercial products such as rice cakes. However if you decide to be grain free then rice of any sort is off the menu.

Cornmeal – Try to ensure that you avoid GM corn by buying organic. Cornmeal is the whole grain unlike cornstarch or cornflour (the UK equivalent). It contains a good source of magnesium, phosphorus, and potassium. In addition it has some B vitamins including B6, niacin and thiamine. This is particularly good flour for cornbread but can also be used in blended flour mixtures (no more than 25%)

Mortina- is an Indian rice grass that is high in protein and fiber. It is made into a flour that adds texture and taste to any mixture of gluten free flour. As mortina also has a strong flavor care needs to be taken not to add too much to avoid overpowering the flavor of the finished product.

Oats (as long as they are labeled gluten free). Oatmeal is particularly high in a fiber called beta glucan. Studies have shown beta glucan to be very effective in lowering cholesterol levels as well as enhancing the immune system. Oatmeal also contains protein.

Sorghum – is a grain that originated in Africa and is rich in iron and fiber. It is increasingly appearing in gluten free flour recipes and has been used to make gluten free beer.

Teff – is a nutritious, ancient grain that originally came from Ethiopia. It is a powerhouse of nutrition with a high protein content. It also contains calcium, thiamine and iron. As well as being used as a flour teff can be fermented and used to make a type of sourdough flatbread. It is best not to use more than 25% in any flour blend due to the fact that it can overpower the flavor.

ALTERNATIVE SEEDS

Buckwheat – is NOT a wheat product despite its name. It isn't even classed as a grain as it is a fruit seed related to sorrel and rhubarb. It is an excellent source of magnesium making it an invaluable food for cardiovascular health and also for controlling blood sugar levels. It can be used as a cereal (flakes) a seed or as a flour.

Millet –is another "grain –like" product that is actually a seed. It is particularly valuable to the body as it is an alkaline food that acts a prebiotic. It provides a variety of nutrients including magnesium, calcium, B vitamins and tryptophan. It is also high in fiber and can be purchased as a seed or as a cereal (flakes).

Quinoa – (pronounced keen-wah) is yet another grain-like seed that is related to the spinach family. It is a complete protein containing all of the essential amino acids needed for body building. It also contains magnesium, manganese, copper and fiber. It is generally cooked as a seed but can also be used as a cereal if bought as quinoa flakes. It is also possible to make it into a flour (see recipe section).

Tapioca – is a starch that many of us may remember as tapioca pudding. It is derived from the root of the cassava plant. It is often used in gluten free flour combinations to add a smoother texture. On its own it has little nutritional value.

OTHER INGREDIENTS THAT CAN BE USED AS FLOURS

Almond Meal or Flour You can grind the almonds whole in a coffee grinder, this is known as almond meal. Alternatively you can blanch the almonds first to remove the skins, this is what we know as almond flour or ground almonds, more popularly used to make marzipan

Arrow Root -This highly digestible starch is made by drying the root of the plant and grinding it into a powder. It contains calcium ash and trace sea minerals

Coconut Flour - This flour is made from fiber that is left once the coconut milk has been extracted from the coconut meat. It is high in fiber and contains small amounts of iron and a trace of sodium

Gram Flour (from chick peas) You can buy gram flour readymade but you may wish to make your own

1. Process 250g dried chick peas in a food processor
2. Sift out any pieces that didn't process and grind in a coffee grinder
3. Sift again to remove any bits and store in an airtight container

Potato Flour - this is made from potatoes that have been cooked, dried and ground and I would advise you to buy a commercial variety rather than try to make this yourself (unless of course you have a dehydrator)

All of these flours are gluten and grain free.

NB - All gluten free flours are best when blended as they add different tastes and textures to the finished product.

I have read comments from people who are looking to start a gluten free diet that most recipe books include products they have never heard of and which they can't buy locally. I am sure that maybe true, but if you want to embrace a healthy gluten free diet then you need to educate yourself regarding these alternative products and include them in your diet otherwise your diet will be severely restricted. If you can't buy them locally then you will inevitably be able to buy them online. I buy several food items online that I can't buy locally with no problems at all. You can put a search into Google or try an Amazon site in your part of the world.

CHAPTER 4
ARE ALL GLUTEN FREE FOODS HEALTHY ALTERNATIVES?

෴

In the early days of being gluten free I used to make good use of the various gluten free products I found on the shelves of the supermarket. However as time has gone by I have started to realize how unhealthy some of these products are. Remember that gluten free doesn't automatically mean it is a healthy alternative. Eliminating gluten may be a healthy choice on the one hand, but the gluten free alternatives available in the health food stores and supermarkets need careful scrutiny before we purchase.

It is important to be aware that the typical western diet is not altogether a healthy diet in the first place and if we simply eliminate gluten and replace it with a gluten free product without making any other changes, our diet will not have improved at all. If you had a diet that contained bread, cakes and biscuits before you were diagnosed the chances are that after you are diagnosed you will simply eat gluten free bread, cakes and biscuits. If you want to heal your gut and repopulate it with good bacteria then you will have to make some more challenging changes to your way of eating.

Many gluten free foods are made with high starch flours such as tapioca, cornflour, and white rice flour etc that have a high glycemic index (GI). The GI is a measure of how quickly a particular food causes blood sugar levels to rise. Potentially they can be responsible for causing hypoglycemia (low blood sugar) caused by sudden rises in blood sugar levels followed by a sudden drop. High GI foods can also be a cause of insulin sensitivity when the body is unable to regulate the amount of insulin it produces and therefore is unable to regulate the amount of glucose in the bloodstream.

To put the Glycemic Index into context, High GI is 70 or above, medium GI is 59 -69 and low GI is 55 or less. We should aim most of the time to have low GI foods, having medium GI foods occasionally and high GI foods only once in a while

Xanthan gum, present in many gluten free products, has been found to induce flu like symptoms in some individuals as well as have laxative properties and being slightly irritating to the gut. There are alternatives that you can use in your gluten free cooking that have the same effect, for example psyllium powder is a good alternative to use in gluten free bread making

A lot of gluten free companies are jumping on the bandwagon by titillating the taste buds with gluten free cakes and biscuits. These products are made with refined gluten free flours and have sugar and other unhealthy sweeteners added, that will do nothing to improve your health. The high sugar content of these products will feed the bad bacteria in the gut which will only serve to exacerbate the individual's health problem.

Inevitably the high carbohydrate and high sugar content will increase the calorific content of the gluten free diet.

Commercial gluten free products are also expensive and are certainly unhealthy for your weekly budget.

Here is a list of ingredients found in the biscuits of a popular gluten free brand

> Sugar, Coconut (27%), Glucose Syrup, Egg White, Dextrose, Potato Starch, Vegetable Oil, Fat Reduced Cocoa Powder (2%), Stabilizer: Sorbitan Tristearate, Emulsifier: Soya Lecithin

Not only does this product contain sugar but it also contains glucose syrup, dextrose a high Glycemic Index monosaccharide(single sugar) and potato starch. The glycemic Index of these products is as follows:-

- Dextrose 100
- Glucose Syrup 100
- Potato Starch 95
- Sugar 70

Here is another list of ingredients for a different popular biscuit product (gluten free)

Orange Jelly (54%); Gluten Free Sponge Biscuit (29%); Chocolate Coating (17%). Orange Jelly contains: Sugar, Glucose Syrup, Water, Natural Flavouring, Gelling Agent: Pectin; Orange Juice from Concentrate, Acidity Regulator: Trisodium Citrate; Citric Acid, Preservative: Potassium Sorbate; Orange Oil. Gluten Free Sponge Biscuit contains: Soya Flour, Sugar, Egg, Maize Flour, Potato Starch, Oligofructose, Glucose Syrup, Raising Agents: Ammonium Hydrogen Carbonate, Disodium Diphosphate, Sodium Hydrogen Carbonate, Soya Oil, Salt, Preservative: Potassium Sorbate; Citric Acid, Maltodextrin, Natural Vanilla Flavouring, Natural Flavouring. Chocolate Coating contains: Sugar, Cocoa Mass, Cocoa Butter, Emulsifier: Soya Lecithin.

Again sugar, glucose syrup, potato starch, maltodextrine are in the list of ingredients

Of course these are sweet products and so will inevitably have some form of sweetener. but they also contain refined flours such as maize flour and soya flour that are also going to be high GI foods. These foods are not going to help towards healing the gut of gluten sensitive people.

So as not to appear to be picking on sweet biscuits, here are the ingredients for a gluten free crispbread.

Rice flour, maize flour, sugar, salt, color: caramel

Again there are 2 flours with a high Glycemic Index and in addition sugar with a GI of 70

Having followed several gluten free blogs and facebook pages I have been surprised to see that even on sites where home cooking is encouraged, the majority of the recipes promoted are of the desserts, cakes and cookies

15

variety. Very little attention seems to be given to the nutritious, healthy, savory gluten free dishes that can be prepared at home. Although I understand why this might be the case, as I know many people love their desserts and puddings, however I also feel that there are far healthier desserts that can be made without the need to add refined sugar and flour. Remember that a healthy gut will not thrive if we continually feed the bad bacteria with sugar. Instead we need to encourage the good bacteria and make wholesome meals that will heal the damaged lining of the gut wall. If you are going to continue with desserts and sweet food please make sure you are using acceptable alternatives in your recipes.

I have several healthy sugar free options for you in the recipe section as well as a recommendation for a book that is full of gluten free healthy desserts and snacks using healthier sugar and flour alternatives.

CHAPTER 5
WHAT CAUSES A LEAKY GUT?

ଔଊ

As a reminder, leaky gut occurs when the delicate lining of the gut is damaged, small holes appear and it becomes more porous. As a result foreign particles such as undigested food particles, bacteria, toxins and yeasts, find their way directly into the blood stream.

It is important to remember that gluten is just one of many causes of damage to the gut wall. Other causes include:-

Poor diet - high refined sugar and processed foods
Prescription medications that cause irritation and inflammation
Stress - leads to weak immune system
Yeast overgrowth leads to low levels of good bacteria in the gut- which in turn weakens   the immune system and creates inflammation

As a result of this process the body becomes irritated and inflamed and the following symptoms may be experienced.

SYMPTOMS

- Inflammation in many different areas of the body
- Joint problems
- Allergies and intolerances
- Autoimmune conditions (when the immune system attacks the body)
- Intestinal gas
- Acid Reflux (acid rising in the esophagus)

- Bowel disturbances such as constipation, IBS colitis etc
- Skin irritations
- Fatigue and low energy
- Brain fog/inability to think clearly/memory loss

It is possible that a leaky gut maybe responsible for many more health problems, especially those that are so far unexplained.

The good news is you can do something about it. If you eliminate the cause of the leaky gut then you at least prevent any further damage. Inevitably, as we have discussed, this will mean giving up gluten, but may also require you to improve your diet in other ways. You are what you eat after all and the food you consume on a daily basis will either help to make you healthy or contribute towards you health problems. The choice is yours.

However with regard to people with Celiac disease, unfortunately, in the majority of cases it isn't simply a matter of just eliminating gluten and the gut will heal.

As I mentioned in the preface In 2009 a study followed 465 Celiac suffers, who eliminated gluten from their diets for 16 months. At the end of the 16 months only 8% of the patients had gut tissue resembling that of a healthy person.

The study also showed that 65% of these gluten free celiacs still had inflammation in the gut. It also showed that the patients had poor vitamin status despite being gluten free. This would seem to indicate that although it is essential to eliminate all gluten from your diet it will not automatically result in the gut healing itself. Something else has to happen to help to heal the gut

So to conclude this section you need to:

- Eliminate all gluten from your diet
- Heal the holes that have occurred in your gut wall
- Repopulate your gut with good bacteria
- Improve your body's ability to digest the food you eat

CHAPTER 6
HEALING THE LEAKY GUT

CЗ80

The first thing to do of course is to eliminate gluten containing products from your diet. You also need to eliminate all processed foods, refined sugars and white flour products (even gluten free ones)

Some people can tolerate dairy but if you have reason to believe it is a problem for you regarding digestion, then you will need to eliminate these foods in the early stages. Some people are intolerant to the lactose and or caesin in milk products so you need to be aware if this may be a problem for you

One of the most important substances that your body needs to heal the gut wall is **L-Glutamine**. L-Glutamine is an amino acid required for the integrity of the gut wall. One of the most natural ways to obtain L-Glutamine is by consuming plenty of bone broth. Bone broth contains three key ingredients that will help to heal the gut wall; glutamine, glucosamine and gelatin. It also contains some important minerals including calcium, phosphorus, magnesium and potassium

There are instructions for the correct method of making the broth and ways to use it in your diet in the recipe section later in the book.

You can of course take supplements containing L-Glutamine if you feel that you want to improve your health more quickly, but obviously supplements cost money and I am trying to offer you money saving methods at this stage. Not only that but the bone broth offers you far more than glutamine for your healing journey

Other helpful supplements might include

- Glucosamine
- Slippery Elm
- Marshmallow Root.

Cabbage has been known to be soothing to the GI tract for many years. It offers nourishment to the cell tissues and has been known to help to sooth the effects of stomach ulcers. Fermented cabbage is particularly beneficial to the healing of the gut as we shall see in the next chapter

REPOPULATING THE GUT WITH GOOD BACTERIA

As part of the healing protocol you need to consider taking a good quality probiotic supplement. However you can also have a long term program of including prebiotic and probiotics foods in your diet.

Prebiotics are the fibrous part of the foods we eat that are undigested. Once they reach the colon they stimulate the growth of the probiotic bifidobacteria. Foods that contain prebiotics include Jerusalem artichokes, leeks, onions and cruciferous vegetables such as cabbage Brussels sprouts and kale.

Probiotics are the beneficial bacteria that live in our gut. They should make up 85% of the bacteria in the gut and provide the vast majority of our immune system. Foods that provide us with probiotics are the cultured and fermented foods such as yoghurt, kefir, sauerkraut and other fermented vegetables all of which will greatly increase the good bacteria in the gut and subsequently improve the immune system.

Fermented products can be made at home. I include a recipe for sauerkraut in the recipe section. It is also possible to make your own yoghurt. In fact if you are intolerant to lactose it is advisable to make you own and allow it to ferment for 24 hours to ensure the lactose is completely digested by the fermentation process. Again, I have included a recipe of how to make this at home.

Your gut needs to be populated with a ratio 85% good bacteria and 15% other bacteria. If this ratio gets out of balance, and it can do so very quickly, you need to work hard to restore the balance and replenish the good bacteria.

Ensuring the integrity of the gut wall and populating it with sufficient good bacteria is essential to your health and well being and your ultimate healing

A staggering 80% of our immune system is in the gut so it is essential that we do what we can to maintain the correct balance of good/beneficial bacteria. This balance is also essential to protect us from an overgrowth of other microorganisms in the gut that can cause inflammation and illness.

IMPROVING DIGESTION

This is also a vital part of the healing protocol and improving the balance of micro flora in the gut aids the digestive process. Fermented products such as sauerkraut (fermented cabbage and/or other vegetables) are very beneficial to the digestive process. So as you can see all of these healing processes are very closely interlinked

Adding digestive enzymes and Hcl and Pepsin will also help the compromised gut to improve the digestive process while healing takes place. (Hcl = Hydrochloric Acid - needed for protein digestion in the stomach)

CHAPTER 7
GLUTEN FREE V GRAIN FREE

❧

There are some health professionals who believe that it is necessary to remove all grains not just those containing gluten.

So why should we choose to be grain free rather than just gluten free?

Unfortunately anybody who has a leaky gut that has been damaged by gluten grains is probably suffering from years of damage. Eliminating gluten grains is certainly the first important change that needs to be made as this eliminates the proteins gliadin and glutenin. As we discussed earlier these proteins are part of a group of toxic proteins called prolamines.

However, although eliminating these two prolamines is very helpful, unfortunately it isn't the whole story. Just to remind you, prolamines are virtually impossible for the digestive system to break down into small enough particles for them to be digested and absorbed.

Grains such as corn, oats and rice also contain prolamines that can cause inflammation in the gut, so many nutritionists will advocate eliminating all grains from the diet to enable the gut to fully recover.

Many of the alternative grains also contain phytic acid a substance that blocks the absorption of nutrients such as calcium, magnesium, zinc and iron. Traditionally grains have been soaked or fermented to neutralize the phytates to make the minerals more accessible to the body.

How far you wish to take this information depends entirely on your own personal situation. I know of many people whose conditions have been so bad that they were virtually allergic to every conceivable food. Their quality of life was so impaired that drastic action was necessary.

This may not be the case for you. In my own situation I found that eliminating the gluten grains, cutting right down on the other grains for a period of time and working hard to heal my gut in the way I have described, was sufficient to see big improvements in my health and eliminate most of my symptoms.

From time to time I do eat gluten now and although I have had no ill effects I am very aware of the potential damage I may be causing and so I proceed with caution.

I regularly consume bone broth, I have virtually eliminated refined sugar from my diet and I choose healthy gluten free options 99% of the time. I would say that generally

I have a healthy healing diet. I also take digestive enzymes and probiotics when I feel my body needs them and I eat fermented and cultured foods as part of my diet. So much of this is about listening to your body. If it is complaining, then you need to do something about it.

For some people, the information here won't go far enough. I am referring to those people who, because of the severity of their symptoms have chosen to follow the SCD (Specific Carbohydrate Diet) or the GAPS (Gut and Psychology Syndrome) diet. Both of which have very strict protocols necessary for those whose systems are in a very bad condition.

I am certainly an advocate of both diets and followed the GAPS diet myself in the early days of diagnosis. It is a very restrictive diet to follow but the motivation to continue with it is due to the fact that it helps you to eliminate many of your symptoms in a short space of time. Motivation is often governed by results and this is no exception.

I also have a friend who after 10 years of trying to solve her health problems, found that the GAPS diet was the only diet that gave her any relief from her symptoms. She still follows the protocol the majority of the time now, 4 years later.

If you suffer from debilitating health problems I am sure, like my friend, you will do anything that you can to find a solution. Sticking to the diet is easy when the result is that you are symptom free.

You will find links to both diet protocols in the resources section at the end of the book

Now for some healthy gluten free recipes to heal the gut and to ensure that it remains in a healthy condition.

CHAPTER 8
HEALTHY GLUTEN FREE RECIPES

൚

BREAKFAST

Breakfast can be one of the most difficult meals to prepare for the gluten free diet, as most people rely on either wheat based cereals or toast and marmalade for their breakfast. I believe that most commercial cereals are completely lacking in any real natural nutritional value and that goes for gluten free commercial breakfasts as well. The more processed the food the less the nutritional value.

For many years I made my own granola as I found the commercial variety too sweet. Before I was gluten free I would use oats, but I now use a combination of other flakes and only add oats to the mix if I am sure they are gluten free.

Granola is very versatile and can be used as a topping for smoothies or can be added to muesli and porridge to give it a bit of texture

I have included some recipes for healthy gluten free bread and these can be used as an alternative to cereal and fruit at breakfast time. The bread is best eaten with a savory such as a boiled egg or an omelet but if your sweet tooth gets the better of you from time to time, you can buy sugar free jam sweetened with apple juice. I am not a jam lover and I find that on these occasions peanut butter seems to work well as it is also quite filling. You can also add sliced banana to the top for a really filling breakfast.

Although my recipes avoid sugar, I do on occasions use a little raw or manuka honey as a sweetener as honey has many therapeutic qualities. You may choose not to do this if you find that honey doesn't agree with you. I may also suggest alternatives such as xylitol and coconut sugar for those who have a sweet tooth. Xylitol is thought to be a good choice for those on an anti candida diet.

GRANOLA

Ingredients

2 cups orange juice
1 tablespoon Coconut oil
1 tablespoon butter
Mixture of flakes of choice - added to reach the correct consistency
Buckwheat/Millet/Brown rice/Quinoa
Sunflower seeds
Chopped mixed nuts

Method

1) Put the orange juice butter and coconut oil into a large pan and bring slowly to the boil to melt the fats.

2) Take of the heat and allow to cool for a few minutes.

3) Mix the flakes together .

4) Add the flakes to the ingredients in the pan and mix all them together until they resemble a stodgy porridge

5) If the mixture is very wet add a few more flakes making sure they are coated and not dry.

6) Spread on a greased baking sheet and bake in the oven for 45 mins.

7) Check at regular intervals and break up the mixture as it dries out.

8) Make sure that the edges don't burn. You may need to adjust the oven temperature depending on your oven type.

9) The mixture should be dry and crisp and light golden brown when completely cooked. If some of the granola is still a little moist – turn the oven right down and cook for a little longer.

10) Break up the mixture if needed and allow to cool.

11) Add any other ingredients such as the sunflower seeds, chopped nuts and dried fruit.

12) Break up the granola and store in an airtight container.

Raspberry and Blueberry Smoothie

Ingredients:

Cup of frozen raspberries.
Small handful of frozen blueberries (or other frozen fruit/ berries of your choice).
Rice milk or almond milk or organic/raw milk if you can tolerate dairy.
1 raw organic egg yolk.
1 scoop protein powder (grass fed whey concentrate) (optional).
Tablespoon Goji berries.
Tablespoon granola or mixed chopped nuts.
Ground flaxseeds, hemp seed, chia seeds (mixed).

Method:

1) Put the fruit and protein powder into a mixer.

2) Just cover with milk of choice.

3) Add the egg yolk.

4) Mix in a blender until smooth like ice cream.

5) Pour mixture into a bowl.

6) Sprinkle with goji berries, ground seed mix and granola or nuts.

NB you may wish to add a teaspoon of raw honey as raspberries can be a little tart, especially if you aren't adding protein powder

This is a power packed healthy breakfast that will last you well until lunchtime. If you want to add some fermented foods to this you can add some yoghurt in place of the milk

MUESLI

Ingredients:

Rice flakes (optional).
Millet flakes.
Quinoa flakes.
Buckwheat flakes.
Make up a mixture and keep in an air tight container. I generally use even amounts of rice, millet and buckwheat and half the amount of quinoa mainly due to the price of the quinoa flakes.
1 or 2 chopped dates .
1 or 2 chopped nuts – any variety.
2-3 tsp mixed ground seeds   I use a combination of flax, hemp and chia seeds and I grind then in a coffee grinder as I need them.
Fresh pineapple or sliced banana or fruit of your choice.
Milk (amount and type to taste).

Method:

1) Put 3-4 tablespoons of the mixed flakes into a bowl.

2) Add the dates, nuts and ground seeds as required.

3) Meanwhile heat up the milk and pour over the flakes.

4) Alternatively if you want cold milk you will need to let the muesli stand for a little while to allow the grains to soak up the milk.

5) Cut up a slice of pineapple (or other fruit) and add to the muesli.

6) You may prefer to simply put the pineapple on top as mixing it in can cause the milk to curdle.

The fruit adds sufficient natural sweetness so there is no need to add any other sweetener.

If you are dairy free you can use alternative milks such as rice milk, or almond milk. I personally don't advocate soy milk as I am concerned about the negative evidence against soy.

PORRIDGE

Ingredients:

40 g brown rice flakes/ or millet (o r mixture of flakes)
Pinch salt
Tblsp Flaxseed/hemp meal
Knob of butter
250ml full cream organic/raw milk (or milk alternative)
Tsp raw honey (or natural sweetener of choice eg xylitol or stevia))

Method:

1) Rinse the rice flakes in cold water in a sieve. Put in a bowl and cover with cold water. Leave to stand for 5 minutes.

2) Put the rice flakes, milk, salt and butter in a saucepan. Bring to the boil and simmer gently for 4 – 5 minutes stirring occasionally.

3) Add the flax meal to the porridge.

4) Serve in a cereal bowl.

5) Add a tsp of raw honey (or alternative) and stir in.

BREAD ALTERNATIVES

GLUTEN FREE FLAX BREAD

Ingredients:

1/3 cup of olive oil
1/2 cup of water
1 teaspoon of sea salt
1 tablespoon of xylitol
1 tablespoon of gluten free baking powder
5 eggs
2 cups of ground organic flax seed/linseed (brown or golden)

Method:

1) Preheat the oven to 350 degrees F.

2) Put the ground flax seed, xylitol, sea salt, and the gluten free baking powder in a bowl and mix well.

3) Crack the eggs into a bowl and beat well

4) Add the oil, water and the eggs and mix well. This mixture needs to stand for a few minutes to allow the flax seed to absorb some of the liquid

5) Line a baking tray with greaseproof paper and oil well

6) Pour the batter on to the tray and spread to approximately 1/2 inch thick.

7) Bake in a preheated oven for approximately 15 -20 minutes depending on oven type. Fan ovens tend to take less time so keep checking

8) To check if the bread is done gently depress the top. If it springs back (a bit like a sponge cake) then it is ready

9) Allow to cool on a cooling tray and cut up as desired.

10) Store in a plastic bag in the fridge or in an airtight container.

Gram Flour Flat Bread

Ingredients:

1 cup gram flour
200 ml water
2 tablespoons extra virgin olive oil
Coconut oil for cooking
1/2 tsp sea salt

Method:

1) Put the gram flour into a bowl.

2) Add the water a little at a time and whisk well making sure there are no lumps.

3) Add olive oil and combine.

4) Leave the mixture to stand to allow the batter to thicken.

5) For a variety of taste you can add ingredients such as pepper, rosemary, coriander seeds, garlic etc.

6) Lightly oil a frying pan with coconut oil.

7) Heat the oil slowly.

8) Add a small amount of the batter to the pan - enough to make a thin pancake.

9) Cook until the flat bread begins to set.

10) Toss the pancake or carefully turn and cook for another minute.

It is also possible to cook in the oven 220 C.

1) Put the batter into a shallow tin.

2) Cook for about 30 mins.

ALMOND FLOUR BREAD

Ingredients:

385g almond flour
3 eggs
120g melted butter
1 tsp. baking soda
1 cup yogurt
1/4 tsp. sea salt

Method:

1) Preheat oven 180 C / 350 F.

2) Mix all ingredients together in a food processor.

3) Pour into a small lined and oiled bread loaf tin.

4) Bake for about 45 minutes.

5) Test with a sharp knife. If it comes out clean - it is done.

6) Leave until completely cooled before removing from tin.

NB This may appear to be a very small loaf but because this is made from almond flour you will find it is extremely filling (as well as nutritious) and only needs to eaten a small amount at a time.

BUCKWHEAT SODA BREAD

In view of the fact that gluten free bread tends to have a very high GI (around 90) it is important to find a bread that has a lower GI for regular use. According to Michel Montignac www.montignac.com the glycemic index of buckwheat soda bread is 40 – so a good alternative

Ingredients:

600 g Buckwheat Flour
½ tsp sea salt
1 1/2 tbsp gluten free baking powder
2 tsp psyllium husk powder
1 tsp vinegar
3 tbsp extra virgin olive oil
500 ml organic milk
2 tbsp buckwheat flour for dusting

Method:

Preheat oven to 200°C/Fan180°C/400°F/Gas 6

1) Mix the buckwheat flour, sea salt, gluten free baking powder and psyllium husk powder in a bowl.

2) Combine the milk, vinegar and oil.

3) Add to the flour mixture.

4) Mix well to form a soft dough

5) Prepare the baking tray by sprinkling with approximately half of the extra flour.

6) Spread the remainder of the flour onto a board and knead the dough into the shape you require, then place the dough on the floured baking tray.

7) Bake in a pre-heated oven for approximately 1 hour 20 mins.

8) The bread should be firm to the touch and have cracks in the crust

9) Take the bread out of the oven and allow to cool on a wire rack

FLAX CRACKERS

Ingredients:

1 cup/100g ground flax seed
1/3 cup grated parmesan cheese
1/2 tsp sea salt
1/2 cup water

Method:

Preheat oven to 200 C / 400 F.

1) Mix all ingredients together.

2) Spoon onto greased parchment paper on a cooking tray.

3) Us a spatula to spread the mixture to about 1/8 inch

4) Make sure the edges are the same thickness a the rest to avoid burning

5) Bake for about 15 mins until the center is firm.

6) If it starts to brown too much around the edges remove from oven.

7) Cut into small squares

8) Leave to cool before removing from tray.

SAVORY DISHES

Many savory dishes require the addition of oil or fat of some sort or use them for cooking our sautéing. I prefer to use olive oil if the food isn't to be cooked and coconut oil, butter or ghee (clarified butter for this who are lactose intolerant) for cooking

HUMMUS

Ingredients:

Can of chick peas in water or 150g dried chickpeas soaked over night.
2 cloves garlic.
Tblsp tahini.
Juice of 1 lemon.
100ml extra virgin olive oil.
Sea salt (to taste).
Paprika or cayenne.

Method:

1) Drain chickpeas (keep the water).

2) Put ingredients in a blender and whiz up to form a smooth paste.

3) Add a little water for a more runny consistency (use water from chickpeas).

4) Empty into a small bowl.

5) Sprinkle with paprika or cayenne pepper.

6) Serve with carrot sticks or gluten free crackers.

NB This can also be made by soaking 200g dried chickpeas over night.

If you want a slightly thinner hummus you can add a small amount of bio yoghurt to reach the required consistency.

You can also add various spices for variety.

FALAFELS

Ingredients:

Can Chickpeas in water or 150g (cup) of dried chickpeas soaked in water over night
3 cloves garlic
Large onion
1 1/2 tsp ground coriander
1 1/2 tsp ground cumin
1 tsp paprika
1/2 cup fresh parsley or 2 tsp dried parsley
1/2 tsp gluten free baking powder
Sea salt
Gram or buckwheat flour if necessary
Coconut oil/butter/ghee for cooking

Method:

1) Chop onion and sauté in a little butter until soft

2) Drain the chickpeas and put them in a blender with the onions, garlic, herbs and spices

3) Blend the ingredients to form a gritty paste

4) Add sea salt to taste

5) If the mixture is too wet you can add some gram flour or buckwheat flour until the right consistency is achieved

7) If time allows leave the mixture, covered, in the fridge for a couple of hours . This will help to prevent the falafels from breaking up during cooking

8) Form into small patties

9) If time allows leave the mixture in the fridge for a couple of hours before cooking

10) Fry gently until lightly browned on both sides.

11) The falafels can be served hot or cold with a mixed green salad and coleslaw or a salad of your choice.

NB Many falafel recipes will tell you to deep fry in very hot oil. I am not in favor of high temperature frying. High temperatures cause free radical damage to the fat , also the polyunsaturated fats , are generally the worst fats to cook with because they are easily damaged by high temperatures. More stable fats suggested above such as butter/ghee and coconut oil are less prone to damage and therefore healthier to cook with.

BUTTERNUT SQUASH RISOTTO

Serves 4

Ingredients:

1 large butternut squash
3 tblsp extra virgin olive oil
2 cloves garlic thinly sliced
1 medium onion chopped
50g butter
1 1/2 liters vegetable stock
350g Arborio rice (risotto rice)
150ml white wine
fresh sage leaves
75g grated parmigiano reggiano

Method:

1) Heat oven to 220 c / gas 7

2) Peel the squash and cut into bite sized pieces

3) Toss the squash, garlic and sage leaves in the oil and put into a roasting tin. Put in the oven for 30 - 40 mins or until the squash is soft and starting to color on the outside

4) Make up the stock and put in a pan. Simmer on a low heat.

5) Put 25g butter into a large pan and sauté the onions until soft

6) Add the rice to the pan with the onions and gently fry until transparent

7) Add the wine and stir until totally absorbed

8) Add the stock gradually ensuring it has been absorbed before adding any more.

9) The grains of rice should be plump but not too firm. It should have a creamy consistency. Extra water can be added if necessary

10) When it is cooked take the squash out of the oven. Divide into two portions. Mash one portion and add to the risotto rice.

11) Add the remainder of the butter and the grated cheese.

12) Serve with the remainder of the squash scattered on top

KEDGEREE

Serves 4

Ingredients:

3 medium organic eggs
350g meaty cod fillets (skinless and boneless) * see below
1 fresh bay leaf
1 yeast-free vegetable stock cube
225g (8oz) of brown basmati rice
1 large knob of dairy and gluten-free spread
1 large clove of garlic (peeled and crushed)
1 medium onion (peeled and chopped)
½ teaspoon of ground coriander
½ teaspoon of turmeric
½ teaspoon of ground cumin
½ teaspoon of fenugreek
½ teaspoon of poppy seeds
½ teaspoon of mustard seeds
115g (4oz) of petit pois
1 tablespoon of fresh lemon juice
Sea salt and freshly ground black pepper to taste

Method:

1) In a pan of boiling water, cook the eggs for 10 minutes. Drain, cool then remove shells and chop the egg.

2) In a large pan with a lid, lay the cod fillets and the bay leaf on the bottom.

3) In a jug, make up the stock cube with 1½ pints of boiling water then pour over the fish so it is covered.

4) Cover with the lid and simmer for about 10 minutes until the fish is cooked then remove the bay leaf.

5) Take the cod out of the stock with a slotted spoon and set it aside in a bowl to flake for use later.

6) In a sieve, add the rice. Rinse well with cold water then add the rice to the pan containing the fish stock.

7) Cover and simmer on a low heat, stirring occasionally. Cook for about 25 - 30 minutes until rice is cooked.

8) Brown rice is temperamental, so you can remove the lid at the end so any excess water can evaporate.

9) Alternatively, you can pour in a little more boiling water, if necessary, to cook the rice for longer until done.

10) In a wok or separate pan, heat the spread. Add the onion and garlic. Stir-fry on a low heat for 5 minutes.

11) Stir in the spices, seeds, petit pois and lemon juice. Then add this together with the fish and the egg to the pan.

12) Warm through and garnish with a sprinkling of freshly chopped chives.

This is a recipe from **Candida Can Be Fun by Rebecca Richardson**

http://www.amazon.com/Candida-Can-Fun-Rebecca-Richardson/dp/0948808144

* The recipe uses unsmoked fish because smoked products are discouraged on an anti candida diet. However it is fine for you to substitute the white fish for naturally uncolored smoked fish if that is your preference

 Rebecca's book can be bought on Amazon via the link above - there is also a link to her website in the resources section

Minty Lamb Burgers

Serves 4

Ingredients:

500g organic lamb mince
I large onion
2 cloves garlic
1 egg
4 teaspoons mint sauce
Sea Salt
Ground black pepper

Method:

1) Chop onion finely and sauté until tender

2) Mix lamb mince and onions together.

3) Add crushed cloves of garlic

4) Add mint sauce

5) Add beaten egg

6) Mix well.

7) Form into small patties

8) Fry gently on both sides in butter or coconut oil until the meat is thoroughly cooked.

9) Serve with mixed salad, coleslaw and potato wedges

FISH CHOWDER

Serves 4

Ingredients:

1 ¾ lb mixed fish pieces (salmon/ white fish/ smoked fish/prawns)
10 oz diced potatoes
3 sticks celery
1 Large or 2 small leeks
Organic crème fraiche
Parsley
Bay leaf
Vegetable stock (gluten free bouillon powder)

Method:

1) Cut up leeks and celery and fry gently in butter or ghee

2) Dissolve vegetable bouillon (gluten free) in 1 pint water

3) Add vegetables, bay leaf and potatoes to the stock and bring to the boil. Boil for 10 mins

4) Cut up fish and add to the pan (not prawns)

5) Cook for further 5 mins to cook the fish.

6) Add prawns and chopped parsley

7) Cook for 2 mins

8) Add 2 tablespoons crème fraiche just before serving

Lentil Shepherd's Pie

Serves 4

Ingredients:

1 cup green lentils
1 large onion
3 stalks celery
3 medium carrots
2 cloves garlic
Herbs eg thyme, rosemary
Vegetable bouillon (gluten free)
2 tablespoons organic tomato paste
Potatoes
Grated Cheese

Method:

Preheat oven 200 C 400 F

1) Chop onion celery and carrots finely. Sauté in butter and leave to sweat in covered pan until soft.

2) Prepare potatoes and bring to the boil

3) Add ½ pint bouillon stock

4) Add lentils and tomato paste.

5) Simmer slowly until the lentils are soft.

6) Add extra water if necessary

7) Add herbs

8) Add crushed garlic and mix well

9) Mash potatoes with a little butter and pepper

10) Put lentil mix in a casserole and cover with mashed potatoes

11) Cover the potatoes with grated cheese

12) Bake in the oven for 15 – 20 mins till golden brown

HERMOULA HALOUMI WITH QUINOA SALAD

This recipe comes from the **India Times**. Time: 1 hour. Serves: 4

Ingredients:

For the Chermoula Haloumi

2 tbsps olive oil (you can use an alternative if you prefer)
1 pkt Haloumi
80 g coriander, including stalks, finely chopped
1 tsp cumin, toasted and powdered
1 tsp paprika
A pinch red chilli flakes
2 lemons, juice only
6 cloves garlic, chopped fine

For the salad:

80 g quinoa
2 lemon, juice only
3 tbsp extra virgin olive oil
4 tbsp chopped coriander
4 tbsp chopped parsley
4 tbsp chopped mint
½ cup pomegranate arils
½ cup mixed peppers chopped fine
Lemon wedges, to serve

Method - For the Chermoula:

1) Put the coriander, cumin, paprika, chilli, lemon and garlic in a blender and blitz, slowly add the oil until smooth.

2) Season with salt, before covering the Haloumi in this marinade.

Leave the Haloumi to marinate for at least 1 hour.

47

For the Quinoa Salad:

1) Cook Quinoa by boiling it double the quantity of salted water or stock for about 10 minutes until it appears to have sprouted.

2) Drain well and tip into a large mixing bowl.

3) Stir in the lemon juice, a splash of the extra virgin olive oil and plenty of salt and pepper.

4) Set aside to cool. When cool add the herbs, peppers and pomegranate to the quinoa and chill.

To cook the Haloumi:

1) Heat 1 tbsp olive oil in a nonstick pan.

2) Add the haloumi and stir-fry until golden and crispy.

To serve

1) Pile the quinoa salad onto 2 plates and place some Haloumi on each mound.

2) Drizzle over a little of the pan juices and serve.

DESSERTS

STEWED FRUIT CRUMBLE

Serves 4-5

Ingredients - For the crumble:

1/2 cup walnuts
1/2 cup almonds
6 pitted dates
1/2 cup shredded coconut (desiccated coconut can be used)
1/4 teaspoon pure vanilla extract
Pinch of salt

Method:

1) In a food processor, chop all ingredients together into a crumbly, but moist texture and set aside in a bowl.

Ingredients - For the stewed fruit:

3 large cooking apples
2 cups frozen berries (raspberries/blackberries etc)

Method:

1) Peel, core and chop the apples, and stew in a little water.

2) Allow the fruit to "fall" so that it is like apple sauce.

3) Add the frozen berries, mix well and put into a casserole dish.

5) Cover with the crumble topping.

This crumble doesn't require any further cooking but it can be warmed in the oven if you prefer.

Fresh Fruit Crunch

Serves 4 -5

Ingredients:

1/2 Fresh medium pineapple
2 cups mixed berries, fresh or frozen (organic if possible)
I large or 2 small organic bananas

Topping:

1 cup muesli mix (see breakfast recipes)
4 chopped dates
2 chopped dried apricots
1 cup mixed chopped nuts
2 oz unsalted organic butter cut into small pieces

Method:

Preheat oven 180 C / 360 F

1) Cut the fruit into bite sized chunks and spread evenly in a shallow casserole dish.

2) Put the muesli mix and the butter into a mixer and pulse on high speed to create fine breadcrumbs.

3) Add the chopped dates, apricots and nuts mix in well to create a crumble topping.

4) Spread the crumble topping over the fresh fruit and bake the oven for 20 mins or until the crumble is slightly crisp and golden in color.

RASPBERRY AND BANANA ICE CREAM

Serves 3- 4

Ingredients:

2 large ripe frozen bananas
1 cup frozen raspberries
1/2 cup bio active yoghurt

Method:

1) Take the bananas out of the freezer half an hour before required

2) After half an hour cut up the bananas and put into a high speed blender with the raspberries and the yoghurt

3) Blend until the banana and raspberries have the texture of ice cream

4) Scoop into individual dishes and top with chopped nuts/goji berries/granola

5) Eat immediately as this cannot be refrozen

Options - grate some organic dark chocolate over the top.

PEANUT BUTTER BISCUITS

Ingredients:

2 ripe bananas
1/3 cup peanut butter smooth or crunchy
1 Large baking apple
I tablespoon vanilla protein powder (optional)
1 tsp vanilla extract
1 1/2 cups muesli flake mixture (see breakfast recipes)
Handful roughly chopped walnuts
1 tablespoons ground flax or hemp seed (2 tablespoons if protein powder not used)

Method:

1) Preheat heat oven to 170°C /350°F. gas 5

2) Stew the apples in a little water and blend to make an apple pulp

3) Mash the banana and combine with the peanut butter.

4) Add the stewed apple, protein powder and the vanilla extract. Mix thoroughly.

5) Add in the oats and the walnuts and mix well.

6) Take a tablespoon full of the mixture at a time and form it into a ball, put on a baking tray (lined with greaseproof/parchment paper) and flatten to make a biscuit shape

7) Bake in the oven for 20 -30 mins.

8) Leave on a cooling tray until completely cold

BANANA BREAD POWER BAR

(Similar to Larabars)

Ingredients:

1/2 cup Medjool Dates
1/2 cup dried banana (described below)
2/3 cup raw almonds

Method:

1) Preheat oven to 175 F 80 C

2) Slice 2 bananas in half and lay them on a greased baking sheet

3) Bake for 2 - 3 hours or until completely dried

4) Alternatively use a dehydrator

5) Combine the dates and dried banana in a food processor and pulse until well combined

6) Remove mixture from food processor and set aside

7) Add almonds to food processor and pulse until a paste forms

8) Add to date and banana mixture and stir well

9) Divide the mixture into 4 equal parts and wrap each in cling film and flatten with a rolling pin

10) Chill in a refrigerator

No Bake Chocolate Oatmeal Cookies

Ingredients:

1/2 cup organic chocolate chips
2 large bananas
1 cup gluten free oats (or buckwheat)
2 tsp vanilla extract
2 tblsp chia seeds
2 tsp raw cacao powder
raw honey to taste

Method:

1) Using a double boiler (or glass dish over a pan of boiling water) melt the chocolate chips stirring constantly

2) Add bananas and stir until well combined

3) Add remaining ingredients and mix well

4) Line a baking sheet with parchment paper

5) Drop by spoonful onto the baking sheet

6) Freeze for one hour or until cookies are firm

Makes about a dozen cookies

The last two recipes are reproduced with permission of the author of *Gleefully Gluten Free (Healthy Desserts and Snacks)* The book is available as an Amazon Kindle book and has lots of healthy dessert recipes. (see resource section)

ALMOND MILK

Almond milk is an ideal substitute for cow's milk if you are dairy intolerant and can be used as alternative in many recipes

Ingredients:

1 cup whole raw organic almonds
Water to soak the almonds
3 cups water for blending

Method:

1) Soak the almonds in water for 12 -24 hours at room temperature.

2) Drain and rinse the almonds.

3) Blend the soaked almonds with 3 cups of water in a food processor.

4) Strain the mixture through fine strainer or cheese cloth

5) The pulp can be reserved for use in other recipes (keep refrigerated)

6) Store your almond milk in the fridge in a sealed glass container for up to 3 days.

You can add a couple of soaked dates to the mixture before blending if you would like the milk to be a little sweeter

Healing Foods for a Healthy Gut

As I mentioned earlier in the book, in order to accelerate the healing of the gut we need to eat large quantities of nutritious bone broth. The bone broth contains glutamine needed for the integrity of the gut wall.

It is the gelatin in the broth that is so healing. If prepared in the correct way the broth also contains many vitamins and minerals including magnesium, calcium, phosphorous and glucosamine. It also contains 2 amino acids called glycine and arganine. Discussing the properties of these nutrients is beyond the scope of this book but suffice to say they have been used to promote health and healing for many years and have been used in Chinese medicine as a boost to the immune system for centuries.

If you are a vegetarian you may not feel this is something that you can do, but unfortunately there isn't really a vegetarian alternative that will have the same effect as the bone broth so depending on the seriousness of your health situation you may have a difficult decision to make.

Avocados also contain some glutamine as do some vegetables and juices, so maybe this would be an option to pursue. As I mentioned earlier you can also take glutamine supplements as an alternative.

In order to make a nutritious broth you will need the following ingredients.

BONE BROTH

Ingredients:

2lb Bones – chicken, beef, lamb or fish
2 tblsp Apple Cyder Vinegar (This helps to draw out the minerals from the bones)
Mixed chopped vegetables (eg onion, garlic, carrot, swede, celery)
Water

Method:

1) Put the bones in a large pan or crockpot (slow cookers are ideal for this)

2) You may need to break up any large bones and may even need to saw them to release the bone marrow.

3) Add the chopped vegetables

4) Cover with cold water

6) Add the Cyder Vinegar

7) Leave to stand for about 30 to 60 mins

8) Bring to the boil

9) Remove the scum from the top and discard

10) Simmer for 6 to 24 hours

11) When cooled strain the liquid

12) For storage you can reduce the liquid by boiling. The broth will then be more concentrated and easier to store

The broth can be kept in the refrigerator for up to 5 days. I generally keep some in the fridge and freeze some in individual glass containers to use whenever I need it.

The broth/stock can then be added to soups and casseroles as required.

A good broth will be gelatinous when chilled.

Ideas For Incorporating Bone Broth

Lamb Cowl

(serves 4)

Ingredients

1 large onion
4 carrots
2 parsnips
Small swede
2 sweet potatoes
4 medium white potatoes
1 oz butter
lamb stock
small pieces of lamb reserved from a roast joint
sea salt

Method:

1) Chop the onion and sauté in the butter until soft.

2) Chop the remainder of the vegetables into mouth-sized chunks.

3) Add to the onions, mix and sauté for about 5 mins.

4) Add the stock plus extra water to cover the vegetables and add a little sea salt.

6) Simmer for 20 mins until the vegetables are cooked. Add additional seasoning if required.

7) Add the lamb and re heat thoroughly.

An alternative to lamb cowl is chicken cowl prepared in the same way but using chicken broth and pieces of chicken in place of the lamb.

It is also possible to use other vegetables but in my experience the root vegetables give the best results.

SOUPS

CARROT SQUASH AND CORIANDER SOUP

Ingredients:

2 medium carrots
1 large slice squash
1 medium onion
stock and water to make up to 1 liter
coriander
2 cloves garlic
1 cup red lentils
sea salt

Method:

1) Finely chop the onion

2) Sauté in a little butter or coconut oil

3) Peel and slice the carrots and squash

4) Add to the onions and cook for a few more minutes.

5) Add the stock and water and bring to the boil

6) Add the red lentils

7) Simmer for approximately 20 mins

8) Add salt to taste

9) Add coriander and crushed garlic cloves

10) Mix in a blender or food processor

11) Serve piping hot with crusty gluten free bread

BROCCOLI AND SWEET POTATO SOUP

Ingredients:

1 onion
1 large or 2 medium sweet potatoes
Half a head of a medium broccoli
Stock and water up to about 1 liter
Sea salt

Method:

1) Chop onion and sauté in a little butter .

2) Peel and chop sweet potato and chop broccoli.

3) Add to onions and sauté over a low heat for about 5 mins.

4) Cover with stock and water and bring to the boil.

5) Simmer for about 20 mins.

6) Add salt to taste.

7) Blend in a food processor.

Options - You can add a handful of red lentils to add some more protein to the soup

These are just two examples of soups I make using the broth. You can add the broth to almost any soup of your choosing

CULTURED AND FERMENTED PRODUCTS

SAUERKRAUT

Another amazing food to help to heal the gut is sauerkraut, included in the diet of some of the healthiest, longest living people in the world. Although cabbage tends to be the most widely used food for sauerkraut you can in fact use many other vegetables either on their own or mixed with cabbage. Whatever you choose the method for making it is the same. However there are in fact a variety of different methods that can used to make sauerkraut and it is up to you to choose one that suits you and works for you. After several disasters I have found the following method, which I consider to be one of the more straight forward methods, to be most successful for me.

Basically sauerkraut is translated as salt cabbage and that is exactly how to prepare it.

Ingredients:

2lb shredded organic cabbage (any sort will do but the harder cabbages are best)
1 tbsp unrefined sea salt
2 cups of filtered water

Method:

1) Shred the cabbage as finely as possible with a sharp knife

2) Put into a large mixing bowl and pound with the end of a rolling pin or a pestle, until the cabbage starts to release its juice

3) Pack tightly into kilner jars leaving space for the added water

4) Mix the salt with the water and pour over the cabbage ensuring the cabbage is well covered and there is approximately ¾" space at the top of the jar

5) Cover with lid and store at room temperature for 3 days, then refrigerate.

CABBAGE AND CARROT SAUERKRAUT

As above but use 1 ½ lb cabbage to ½ lb carrots

You can also add ingredients such as garlic and ginger to produce a different taste

The authority on fermenting vegetables is Sally Fallon who wrote **Nourishing Traditions**, a book I highly recommend.

NB Another popular way of making sauerkraut is the layer cabbage and salt and then pummeling the mixture until it produces enough of its own liquid to cover the cabbage. This method is more difficult to do and in my experience less successful, though I know it is highly recommended by some.

It is also possible to make sauerkraut using a starter that will help the fermentation process.

YOGHURT

Ingredients:

1 liter organic full cream milk (preferably raw)
Commercial yoghurt starter or 2 tblspns plain **bio** yoghurt

Method:

1)Heat the milk to simmering point and then remove from the heat.

2)Allow to cool to room temperature. I use a milk thermometer to ensure it is at the correct temperature

3)Mix the yoghurt with a little milk to make a paste.

4)Add the remainder of the milk and mix well.

5) Pour into a yoghurt maker or wide necked thermos flask.

6)Leave to ferment for 12 hours for normal yoghurt or 24 hours for SCD yoghurt.

NB - a thermos flask may not be sufficient for 24 hour fermentation as the yoghurt will cool down significantly during the longer period of time.

The finished yoghurt can be runnier than commercial yoghurt. If you prefer, you can strain some of the whey off the yoghurt to thicken it. The whey can be used as a starter for sauerkraut in addition to the salt. This adds the probiotic to the sauerkraut to enhance the fermentation process.

CREAM CHEESE

It is also possible to make cream cheese by straining the yoghurt through a cheese cloth until it resembles the right consistency.

Add a little salt and any other flavorings such as herbs and garlic.

ABOUT THE AUTHOR

ଔଓ

My name is Janet Matthews and I am a retired head-teacher of a centre for pupils with emotional and behavioral problems. I have a diploma (Dip ION) in nutritional practice from the Institute of Optimum Nutrition in London in 1988 and have had an active interest in health and personal development for many years.

My other qualifications include:-

Life Coaching Diploma
Enneagram Teacher (part 1)
MBTI Practitioner
Metabolic Typing Practitioner

I have been writing online as a ghostwriter for over 6 years and I have several health related blogs of my own. I have also been a guest writer for other blogs and websites on the subject of health and well- being.

Really Healthy Gluten Free Living is my second book. My first book Is Stress Your Silent Killer? is also available on Amazon.

I have plans for many more in a series of self help, health and wellbeing ebooks, and will post them in the resources section as and when they become available. Alternatively you can visit my website http://your-healthy-options.com for updated information on my books, products and recommendations.

RESOURCES

CR80

I ou would like further information on gluten free living or other health issues you can find me on the following links:-

My website http://your-healthy-options.com

My facebook fanpage http://facebook.com/yourhealthyoptions

I would love to hear your thoughts about this book — feel free to email me at

janet@your-healthy-options.com

Books and websites I recommend

For more information on the grain free protocol for those whose symptoms are more severe and are not clearing up by simply eliminating gluten, I would highly recommend the following books available on Amazon, and their related websites.

Gut and Psychology Syndrome by Dr. Natasha Campbell-McBride

http://www.amazon.com/Gut-Psychology-Syndrome-Depression-Schizophrenia/dp/0954852028/

website - http://www.gapsdiet.com/

Breaking the Vicious Cycle - Elaine Gottschall

http://www.amazon.com/Breaking-Vicious-Cycle-Intestinal-Through/dp/0969276818/

website - http://www.breakingtheviciouscycle.info/

SCD Quick Start Guide (free guide available on the website)

website - http://www.scdlifestyle.com/

Candida Can Be Fun by Rebecca Richardson

website http://www.candidacanbefun.co.uk

FOR MORE INFORMATION ON HOW TO HAVE A COMPLETELY GLUTEN FREE HOME -

Simple Gluten Free Living by John Turner (Amazon Kindle)

http://www.amazon.com/dp/B007I4BHRG

John became gluten free when his wife was diagnosed with Celiac Disease, and has shared in his book what it takes to ensure your home and especially your kitchen are completely Gluten Free

FOR MORE HEALTHY GLUTEN FREE DESSERTS

Gleefully Gluten Free (Healthy Desserts and Snacks) by Ruth Naylor

http://www.amazon.com/dp/B008MNR6JA

Ruth has produced an ebook that will help the gluten free sweet tooth without causing too much harm to the gut. One or two of the recipes may need to have a different natural sweetener if you have a lot of bloating, but the recipes all use the healthiest ingredients possible to satisfy the sweet tooth. As I have said before it is important to listen to your body and respond accordingly.

MY OTHER EBOOKS

Is Stress Your Silent Killer?

http://www.amazon.com/dp/B009KTI1OY/

I have approached this book from the premise that stress can have a detrimental effect on the immune system and ultimately cause life threatening illnesses.

"Having suffered from chronic stress myself, I am only too aware of the detrimental effect this can have on our health and well-being. In this book I will share my own experience, what it taught me about myself, and how, through a deeper inner knowledge, I was ultimately able to begin to stress proof my life."

Janet Matthews (author)

What other have said:

"This is a very well researched and well written book. In this educational read Janet Matthews the author shares her own story of coming through chronic fatigue and her journey back to health. She shares some great insights into the causes and potential cures and preventatives and also talks about the spiritual and emotional healing aspects of stress"

A Fischer (Amazon review)

" I am so thankful to have had the opportunity to read this amazing book! You have helped me to see where I am now, and where I MUST go. I am a chronic stressor and already have health issues, undoubtedly due to stress. I used to practice yoga and some meditation. I have gotten away from this routine, because I "didn't have the time". Because of you and this book I am reminded, that I MUST make the time for me! A MILLION THANKS TO YOU!!!!"

Susan Joseph (via unsolicited email)

MEDICAL DISCLAIMER

☙❧

The contents of this book are provided for informational and educational purposes only. They are not intended to be a substitute for professional medical advice, diagnosis, treatment (including medical treatment), psychotherapy, counseling, or mental health services.

Consult a physician or other qualified health professional regarding any opinions, information or recommendations with respect to any symptoms or medical condition.

Made in the USA
Lexington, KY
17 August 2013